Infrared and red light therapy guide

The ultimate guide to fight aging, improve cognitive function, improve skin, gain muscle, increase athletic, cognitive and brain performance, recover athletically and mentally faster, relieve and control pain from arthritis and other diseases, improve sleep and mental health, help with fat loss and hair loss, as well as improve overall health and wellness.

DAVID BUHNER

RED LIGHT AND INFRARED LIGHT THERAPY GUIDE

Copyright © 2023 DAVID BUHNER

First Edition: January 2023

INDEX

CHAPTER 1

What is red light therapy?

Is therapy using real red and infrared light effective?

Red light and infrared light have emerged as scientific surprises in recent years, highlighting the influence of the intangible on our health. On previous occasions, I have explored the effects of radiation and grounding (being in contact with the earth) as invisible but fundamental elements for wellness. Will red and infrared light earn a place on this list?

The earliest hints of the health benefits of red light in the modern era date back to Endre Mester, a Hungarian physician famous for pioneering laser technology. In distant times, he calibrated one of his lasers while experimenting and unexpectedly opened the belly of a sleeping rat to implant a tumor and then remove it as part of his research.

To his surprise, the laser did not destroy the tumor, but somehow healed the incision. The doctor was perplexed. How could the laser have missed the tumor but healed the wound? This accidental incident revealed the existence of "photobiomodulation" in that rat1J Laser Dent 2009;17(3):146-148, a tissue repair process activated by infrared light.

Endre's laser turned out to be much dimmer than he thought, an experimental accident that highlighted one of the benefits of low-intensity infrared light therapy.

It is important to remember that a laser is nothing more than an amplification of light stimulated by radiation, in fact, the word "laser" comes from its function: Light Amplification by Stimulated Emission of Radiation.

In short, we are talking about light, but not just any kind.

It's not as simple as simply exposing your skin to lights of all colors at any time to revitalize it. Otherwise, our fun nights at the disco could be considered the healthiest decisions in life.

I am addressing a light therapy that, as expected, seeks to emulate probably the most crucial component of nature: the sun.

It is no coincidence that throughout virtually every historical culture (with the exception of our own), our ancestors have revered the sun. We even have photographs from the 1920s that depict wounded soldiers resting outside hospitals.

At the time, nurses opted to place the beds outside, allowing the sun's rays to accelerate wound recovery, according to what the medical community had observed.

Even in the 1930s, some governments distributed pamphlets to families with the title "sunlight for babies," recommending that they take their children outside to get as much exposure to sunlight as possible.
They literally stated: "Every mother who wants her baby to be in good health should expose it regularly to sunlight from infancy until it is old enough to play by itself in the sun".

Although I have addressed the importance of getting vitamin D from the sun, I have recently realized that the sun provides us with much more than just vitamin D.

Our cells are receptive to the various types of light to which we expose them. This applies not only to the light we catch with our eyes, but also to the light that strikes our skin, the largest organ in our body.

•

Even when we close our eyes, our skin continues to perceive not only the presence of light, but also the type of light that is illuminating it. In this way, each exposure to light implies that our body absorbs or "downloads" information.

Some years ago, during a visit to a friend, I was told about the mother of someone they knew, who "nourished from the sun" (...). At the time, I considered it a fanciful tale, but now I realize that perhaps I was the one who judged without giving it due consideration.

I would like to express my special thanks to the members of the private community (especially Sergio Elortegi and Festuc) for addressing these issues in such depth and giving them the importance they deserve.

Treatment with red light or infrared light (NIR)?

Although the visual perception of light is possible for our eyes, we must remember that light is an electromagnetic wave, similar to microwaves, X-rays, infrared or radio waves. Unlike these invisible waves, the peculiarity of light is that it is a visible electromagnetic wave, composed of magnetic and electric fields.

The health impacts of electromagnetic waves, whether positive or detrimental, are a reality. Therefore, we can infer that if certain wavelengths (such as X-rays or microwaves) can have negative effects, other wavelengths, such as light, could also have a positive influence on our health.

It is important to note that while blue light, whether from the sun or artificial sources, stays in the superficial layers of the skin, red light has the ability to completely penetrate our skin, reaching organs and even bones.
A leading expert on the subject with an extensive list of scientific publications is Dr. Michael Hamlin. In his explanations, he addresses in a practical way the concept we have just reviewed.

To illustrate this point in a simple way, we can consider the following example: if we take the flashlight of our cell phone and cover it with our finger, we will observe only a red glow. This is because only red light frequencies are able to pass completely through our finger.

Each of these segments of light, which takes on different colors, performs specific functions and interacts uniquely with the body, telling it how to activate certain mechanisms.

The wavelength of this electromagnetic wave, i.e. light, determines its color. The longer the wavelength, the redder the light, and the deeper it penetrates into the body, even through the bones.

Here arises one of the most common confusions: red light or infrared light? It is important to note that these are two different entities.

What really is infrared light?

Analyzing visible light, we come across an intriguing phenomenon: as the wavelength increases and the light becomes red-tinted, it reaches a point where it is no longer visible to the human eye, becoming infrared light, imperceptible to us.

Solar radiation reaching the Earth includes both visible light and infrared light, the latter being invisible to us. Only a small portion of ultraviolet light reaches us.

Although ultraviolet light has been criticized, it is essential for the production of vitamin D through sun exposure. Nature, always synergistic, reveals that infrared light and its benefits act as a defense against UV light.

You may remember the image of the retired truck driver with one half of his face more wrinkled than the other. The media, in their eagerness to blame the sun, present this as a negative effect.

It turns out that this truck driver spent most of his time under sun exposure, but through the windows of his vehicle. This means that he only received ultraviolet (UV) light and lacked the infrared light that acts as an antioxidant shield. Herein lies the problem: the modern invention of glass that filters out the beneficial from the sun, letting in only the harmful.

In fact, more than 50% of solar energy is infrared. Campfires, fireplaces, candles and incandescent lights also emit infrared light. These were the light emitters our ancestors were exposed to before the advent of LED light.

It was not until recent decades that, at the University of Florence, the numerous anti-aging effects associated with infrared and red light were discovered.

What is actually the red light?

I understand that as you start down the path of understanding about red light therapy, questions arise. What exactly do you mean by light? Are you talking about the end part of visible light, i.e. red light? Or are you talking about the invisible light that is already infrared?

The answer covers both sides.

When "red light therapy" is mentioned, it refers to a light that includes a small portion of visible light (hence we see devices with red light, as it is light that we can perceive), covering a much wider range of infrared light, which escapes our ability to see.

In other words, when we mention "red light therapy", we mean the combination:

- Perceptible red light ranges from 660 nanometers to 700 nanometers.

- Even infrared light, which escapes our visual perception, extends down to 850 nanometers.

It is in this specific range that health benefits have been observed.

While visible red light stimulates various cells to grow, reproduce and contribute to collagen synthesis, near invisible infrared light reduces cell proliferation, favoring the maturation of cells to produce and release collagen.

Thus, all therapies that are labeled as "red light therapy" actually encompass a "two-in-one therapy". In these therapies both types of light are combined.

You may be wondering why not increase the power even further. The reason lies in the fact that, although infrared light extends beyond 850 nanometers, it has been observed that the effective therapeutic range is from 660 to 850 nanometers.

How to perform infrared light treatments?

Lamps designed for home treatments seek to replicate the function of the sun, covering a specific wave range from 660 to 850 nm. Compared to bathtubs or showers, these lamps are a more accessible and convenient alternative for similar benefits. Just as we choose a shower at home instead of plunging into the river or the sea, these lamps offer convenience and accessibility.
There are small, portable models that cover specific areas of the body, while larger, more powerful models cover the entire body, allowing you to choose between general therapy or focus on a specific wavelength for more targeted benefits.

The practice of exposing oneself to the sun for its benefits is not new; the ancient Egyptians practiced "heliotherapy", and Hippocrates, considered the father of modern medicine, prescribed "exposure to sunlight" based on his observations of the benefits of the sun.

The conclusions I drew when I noticed that Greek and southern communities, enjoying more hours of sunshine, exhibited greater happiness and optimism compared to northern populations, were revealing.
During sunrise and sunset, the sun provides us with red and infrared light therapy free of charge, regardless of any device.

•

That is why during the approximately 30 minutes of each sunrise and sunset, we observe reddish tones in the sky. At these times, the sun offers us an additional dose of red light, charged with infrared radiation, which is extremely beneficial for us.

Because of this, the industry has taken on the task of developing devices that mimic this light. Another ruse to sell you something? Well, we can experience this therapy without shelling out a single euro.

What you really need is something our ancestors possessed in abundance (as well as good health): time.

Time to reap the benefits of an ancestral practice that our ancestors enjoyed in good company: sunrises. We can also mention the warmth of campfires (...).

Devices, such as lamps that recreate this light artificially, are useful to emulate the natural sunrise environment if you don't have the time to witness it, or on more cloudy days, or when your location is not conducive to enjoying them. For example, I apply it during the evening while I dilate a bit. I take off my clothes and expose myself to the red light.

However, as in everything in life, moderation is the key.

Just as sunrise and sunset do not occur 24 hours a day, we should not abuse exposure to red light.

The reality, dear followers of life, is that unless you live in a country house (in which case, I envy you), most of us who reside in a city or even a town are not as exposed to red light. Where I live, the sun is hidden behind the buildings to the east, and despite having looked for different locations at 7:20 in the morning in the spring, I have yet to find the perfect spot. I hope to find it soon. For this reason (if you can afford it), I recommend one of these devices.

What are the impacts of red light on the organism?

Our organisms have evolved to allow the absorption of this light, but the underlying mechanism is a matter of controversy. Although it is recognized that there are benefits, we still do not fully understand the chain events that occur. It is similar to understanding that gaining more muscle mass and strength is beneficial, but we do not fully understand how this is achieved. We know the elements necessary to build muscle, such as mechanical tension, metabolic stress, calories and hormones, but the exact steps and mechanism remain unknown.

- Current theory suggests that, during exposure to red light, a cell-stressing molecule called nitric oxide is generated. Through certain processes, this molecule makes it easier for cells to "breathe more".
- Since it is a stress molecule, small amounts of free radicals are generated.
- This promotes vasodilation, related to nitric oxide and of great importance in situations of inflammation, such as swollen joints (which is why red light is beneficial for arthritis).

- Red light therapy also affects the water present in the cells, generating a greater separation between water molecules. In practical terms, we are altering the physical properties of the cell, reducing the resistance between enzymes and proteins, which facilitates the more efficient occurrence of cellular reactions.

This phenomenon is not only limited to the interior of cells, but also impacts the blood and intercellular spaces.

The complexity of life, even at the cellular level, is not fully understood, but what we do know is that red and infrared light therapy plays a key role in vitality. However, most of us are deficient in this area.

From a biological perspective, although we do not fully understand the mechanism, we could summarize that exposure to red light affects cells, driving them in one of three directions: [here you should add specific information about the directions].

- Cells, during exposure, will follow one of two paths: self-repair if damaged or self-destruct if necessary.

- Thanks to a greater supply of energy, with an increase in ATP, the cell will undergo a kind of evolution, becoming more efficient in its functions.

- When we are exposed and the concentration of cells in that region is reduced, a stimulus is produced that favors the migration of more cells to that area or induces their growth.

How does the red light benefit us?

Currently, there is an extensive database with thousands of research studies on photobiomodulation, a state our body enters to begin to experience health and anti-aging benefits through red light therapy and near infrared light therapy. You can find more information about these studies at this link: [Photobiomodulation Research Database] (https://docs.google.com/spreadsheets/d/1ZKl5Me4XwPj4YgJCBe s3VSCJjiVO4XI0tIR0rbMBj08/edit#gid=0).

In fact, all the benefits we derive from the various branches and functions of our body can be summed up in one word: mitochondria.

When we talk about more efficient mitochondria, we are referring to the specialized equipment that works tirelessly to provide the energy necessary for life. In the human body, this energy, known as ATP, is essential for our cells to carry out their inherent processes.

Imagine these "ATP janitors" as the gatekeepers who hold the master key to all cellular doors. They reside in the mitochondria, the nuclear powerhouses of our cells, or we could call them the powerhouses of these janitors. The more mitochondria we have, the more janitors we are equipped with, which translates into the ability to open doors and activate bodily functions more quickly and efficiently.

The more of these cellular nuclear power plants called mitochondria we have, the more energy we can generate.

One way to increase the amount of mitochondria is through exercise. That is why athletes have more mitochondria in their muscles compared to sedentary people[5].

However, a dilemma arises when focusing on simply increasing the number of these janitorial power plants, i.e., mitochondria. The goal is not just to have a team of janitors, but to make sure that they are young and efficient. There is no point in creating more and more mitochondria if they end up being slow and inefficient. What is the point of having a large number of mitochondria if they are old, slow and inefficient in opening doors and activating cellular functions? The ideal is to have a team of mitochondria in optimal condition. And what better way to keep them young and healthy than by exposing them to sunlight every day? Specifically, to that solar infrared light.

Some scientists have begun to call this process "human photosynthesis". Just as plants obtain energy from the sun to carry out their processes, humans need this solar radiation so that the mitochondria, those nuclear power plants linked to our cells, produce the necessary ATP energy: the efficient conservers.

Additional power generation.

ATP plays the crucial role of overseeing all biological processes in the body. These "janitors" must not only open doors quickly (i.e. facilitate all processes in every cell), but it has also been observed that ATP is used for communication between cells.

In short, if you suffer an injury, these "janitors" are responsible for transmitting the message to the cells in charge of repairing the damage. The more inefficient, older or clumsier your "janitor" equipment is, the longer it will take to transmit this message and the longer it will take for the muscle tissue to repair itself, as it will depend on how fast your energy, your ATP (i.e. the "janitors"), is working.

In addition, efficient communication between the various parts of the body contributes to protection against neurodegenerative diseases, thus promoting a stronger state of health.

.

- People with type 2 diabetes face the challenge of having a pancreas that does not operate optimally. Low energy production is recorded in pancreatic mitochondria, according to studies6Haythorne, E., Rohm, M., van de Bunt, M. et al. Diabetes causes marked inhibition of mitochondrial metabolism in pancreatic β-cells. Nat Commun 10, 2474 (2019). An essential organ for insulin production when required. Furthermore, when insulin resistance is present in cells, energy generation in mitochondria is reduced7Szendroedi, J., Phielix, E. & Roden, M. The role of mitochondria in insulin resistance

.

and type 2 diabetes mellitus. Nat Rev Endocrinol 8, 92-103 (2012).

- In Parkinson's disease, the evidence is compelling for the crucial role of mitochondria8Wright, R. Mitochondrial dysfunction and Parkinson's disease. Nat Neurosci 25, 2 (2022).

- In the case of Alzheimer's disease, one of the characteristic pillars of this disease is, as you might have guessed, reduced energy production in the mitochondria9Mary, A., Eysert, F., Checler, F. et al. Mitophagy in Alzheimer's disease: Molecular defects and therapeutic approaches. Mol Psychiatry 28, 202-216 (2023).

Improving the health of your mitochondria is tantamount to improving your overall well-being. It starts by protecting your brain against neurodegenerative diseases like Parkinson's and Alzheimer's, but the brain benefits of healthier mitochondria don't stop there.

Decreases levels of sadness and worry.

Remarkable improvements in depression and anxiety symptoms have been observed with infrared and red light therapy. It all started with small studies more than a decade ago, and have recently been replicated and resumed. To sum it up... they improved (Schiffer et al., 2008).

In as little as 4 weeks, 60% of patients were in remission, with fewer depressive symptoms, and 70% reported feeling almost no anxiety. It was at this point that light therapies began to be taken seriously for mental health (Cassano et al., 2016).

Initial studies involved depressed rats exposed to stressful situations, and those that received infrared light therapy showed reduced hormonal responses, especially cortisol, the stress hormone.

The research then moved to more recent human studies. A particularly striking one was conducted in 2017 with 39 patients with depression, where after 16 weeks, 32 of them experienced complete or near-complete remission of depression (Henderson & Morries, 2017). Furthermore, the mental benefits were observed to persist for an average of 55 months after the end of the study.

Although depression has multiple factors, improvements are not surprising. Personally, after living in several places, including Sweden, Estonia, Canada and Finland, I can attest to the importance of sunlight on well-being.

Historically, no indigenous tribe has existed without exposure to the sunlight in their environment. While the word "cure" may be risky, it is undeniable that improvements do occur. The proliferation of studies may be driven by economic interests, as industry sees the potential to sell expensive lamps and devices. However, those of us here know that enjoying sunset and sunrise can offer similar benefits, which, by the way, are not limited to these aspects alone.

Increases testosterone generation and sexual desire.

In my therapy sessions at home with sunlight using lamps (since I cannot do it outdoors yet), one of the practices I do is to expose myself completely.

This choice is based on observations of improvements in testosterone levels in the 635-670 nanometer range. An excuse to stop consuming bull cryadillas? Perhaps it is better to opt for both?

It makes sense that exposure to red light raises testosterone levels, also from an evolutionary perspective. In the northern hemisphere, testosterone decreases during the winter months, probably due to the lack of light. This theory is further strengthened by observing how testosterone increases again as spring and summer approach.

Why would nature follow this pattern? To encourage proliferation and increase the chances of hatchling survival. As mentioned above, there tends to be more offspring in late August, when there is more sunshine and months of abundance, which ensures that the mother is loaded with vitamins and the baby is born in the spring, with access to more food and light for the parents.

In the infrared light studies, men with low sexual interest were used as subjects, and it was confirmed that this light increased their libido and testosterone. An increase was also observed in rats, although in some cases, exposure to red light was detrimental to their reproductive organs.

Does it make sense that testosterone increases with certain light ranges? Nature is guiding us hormonally, with more or less libido, towards the best times to have offspring.

In my case, I risk doing my sessions in balls, but since this is not nutritional advice, the choice is up to you. To me, it makes sense that anything that, with common sense, would not harm other areas and tissues, could also be beneficial for these little guys we have between our legs.

An increase in collagen production is observed, which contributes to improved skin quality.

Moving into the realm of specific areas, there is one sector where monetary investment is quite common, especially among women: skin care. And, as you might have deduced, this care also experiences remarkable improvements with red light therapies.

•

I came across a particular study that focused on women with melasma, a hyperpigmentation condition that results in the appearance of dark areas on the face. These women were subjected to infrared therapy, but with an interesting twist: the lights were applied to only one part of the face. The end result (pay attention) was that at the conclusion of the study, there were improvements not only in that specific area, but in the entire face in general.

This is because there is an abundance of evidence supporting how red light promotes collagen synthesis18Illescas-Montes, R., Melguizo-Rodriguez, L., Garcia-Martinez, O. et al. Human Fibroblast Gene Expression Modulation Using 940 NM Diode Laser. Sci Rep 9, 12037 (2019).19Pérignon, B., Bandiaky, O.N., Fromont-Colson, C. et al. Effect of 970 nm low-level laser therapy on orthodontic tooth movement during Class II intermaxillary elastics treatment: a RCT. Sci Rep 11, 23226 (2021).20Koorman, T., Jansen, K.A., Khalil, A. et al. Spatial collagen stiffening promotes collective breast cancer cell invasion by reinforcing extracellular matrix alignment. Oncogene 41, 2458-2469 (2022).21Yeh, MC., Chen, KK., Chiang, MH. et al. Low-power laser irradiation inhibits arecoline-induced fibrosis: an in vitro study. Int J Oral Sci 9, 38-42 (2017).22Hwang, M.H., Son, H.G., Lee, J.W. et al. Photobiomodulation of extracellular matrix enzymes in human nucleus pulposus cells as a potential treatment for intervertebral disk degeneration. Sci Rep 8, 11654

(2018).23Kang, M.H., Yu, H.Y., Kim, GT. et al. Near-infrared-emitting nanoparticles activate collagen synthesis via TGFβ signaling. Sci Rep 10, 13309 (2020)....

Collagen is an essential protein that forms the basis of our connective tissue. Without healthy collagen, it is difficult to maintain good condition in areas such as hair, skin, nails, joint health, muscle growth and even brain cognition. This is why improvements are seen in various indicators, such as depression (as has been observed), arthritis (a condition that affects the joints), skin health, among others.

It is not surprising that the marketing of collagen supplements has experienced a considerable increase in the last decade, exposing a negative facet of capitalism: unknowing consumption. We refer to a staggering figure of 500 billion (in the case of this supplement alone).

There is no need to resort to a collagen supplement if you understand some basic health concepts. What is truly essential is the collagen that is naturally found in the body, not in supplement form. We need it to obtain the very thing that this magnificent podcast of knowledge provides us with: proper synthesis, and with the application of red light, the benefits are remarkable.

•

After observing how collagen production in wounded animals significantly accelerated healing24Biostimulation of wound healing by lasers: experimental approaches in animal models and in fibroblast cultures - R. Abergel, R. Lyons, +2 authors, we began to apply this approach in humans. Using ranges from 622 to 830 nanometers, wrinkle visibility was reduced in participants after 12 weeks25Russell, B. A., Kellett, N. & Reilly, L. R. A study to determine the efficacy of combination LED light therapy (633 nm and 830 nm) in facial skin rejuvenation. J. Cosmet. Laser Ther.7, 196-200.

You might think, "this is just a gimmick to get women of a certain age to buy red light bulbs in the teleshop," but randomized studies have been conducted with placebo and double-blind groups. It doesn't get any more scientific than this....

And what does the outcome tell us? A 36% decrease in wrinkles and a 19% increase in skin elasticity after undergoing biweekly treatment26A prospective, randomized, placebo-controlled, double-blinded, and split-face clinical study on LED phototherapy for skin rejuvenation: clinical, profilometric, histologic, ultrastructural, and biochemical evaluations and comparison of three different treatment settings. Seung Yoon Lee, Ki-Ho Park, +6 authors.

It provokes an antioxidant reaction in the organism.

When we experience an increase in energy thanks to the stimulation of red light, what happens is that the cells choose to absorb more oxygen, generating reactive oxygen species, that is, the so-called free radicals that industry has insisted we fear, such as those coming from the sun.

However, it is important to note that exercise also leads to the production of free radicals, as does exposure to cold and sun. In fact, simply being alive already involves some level of exposure to these elements.

Why would we look to our cells to cope with stress? Well, as nature dictates, "if you don't use it, you lose it". By subjecting cells to occasional stress (to a small extent), we end up obtaining therapeutic benefits.

Optimizes sleep quality indicators.

When we expose ourselves to infrared light from the sun or devices designed for this purpose, nitric oxide production is also increased. This compound is used by bodybuilders as a supplement to dilate blood vessels, thus achieving greater muscle engorgement

•

during and after training, giving the appearance of greater size temporarily.

What many gym-goers are unaware of is that nitric oxide, having a vasodilator effect, lowers blood pressure, increases flow, relaxes muscles, calms the body, and decreases respiratory rate. Put another way, it seems to signal that it's time to go rest. It turns out that this red light therapy also contributes to sleep, and one of the main factors for this to occur is precisely the nitric oxide generated[27]Gautier-Sauvigné, S. et al. Nitric oxide and sleep. Sleep Med. Rev. 9, 101-113 (2005)....

But the positive influence is not only limited to nitric oxide, it also affects the regulation of melatonin, known as the sleep hormone, which is in charge of controlling our sleep-wake cycles. As I mentioned in some episode of the podcast, melatonin not only induces sleep, but acts as a sort of guide. It signals the body that it's time to sleep, but its function goes beyond that.

Research on melatonin regulation after red light therapy sessions has increased[28]Morita, T. & Tokura, H. Effects of lights of different color temperature on the nocturnal changes in core temperature and melatonin in humans. Appl. Human Sci. 15, 243-246 (1996).[29]Red light and the sleep quality and endurance performance of Chinese female basketball players. Zhao J, et al. J Athl Train. 2012. PMID: 36830774 Free PMC article. Clinical

Trial. and as expected, the industry has marketed melatonin as a star supplement.

In reality, when someone experiences difficulty falling asleep, it is often related to the disconnection from light, with the lack of "solar information downloading" at the right time. There is a solid argumentation behind this:

We should produce melatonin instead of "taking" it. Just as we generate vitamin D in our skin when we expose ourselves to the sun, instead of "taking" it.

In the body, we find two forms of melatonin: circulatory (produced in the pineal gland) and subcellular (produced within cells and mitochondria). Melatonin not only dictates bedtime, but also exerts significant protection over our brain, acting as a kind of overprotective mother figure.

It is surprising to note that approximately 45% of people with Alzheimer's disease or dementia suffer from the so-called sunset syndrome. From the name alone, we can already infer that daylight hours and mental health are closely linked and should not be taken lightly.

Sunrise and sunset do not receive the attention they deserve. Cognitively ill people who experience sunset syndrome become significantly agitated. Their brains do not recognize the time of day and it has been speculated that this is due to minimal melatonin levels30Khachiyants, N., Trinkle, D., Son, S. J. & Kim, K. Y.

•

Sundown syndrome in persons with dementia: An update. Psychiatry Investig. 8, 275-287....

Why wouldn't you want more melatonin through infrared therapy? Or rather, why wouldn't you want to have more at the right time? We want our mother to be present in our lives, but not in every moment of our daily activities. We do not want her in the bathroom while we take care of our physiological needs, nor when we share the bed with our partner.... Is that understood? Melatonin is essential, but it is even more crucial that it fulfills its function at the right time.

If we lack light, it will be the pineal gland that will be in charge of generating melatonin, but the most effective stimulus for subcellular melatonin comes from infrared light. Lamps can be useful, but nothing compares to natural sunlight.

Specifically, non-visible infrared light reaches all parts of the body, penetrating completely, including the skull and accessing the cerebrospinal fluid. This further reinforces the reason why people with neurodegenerative diseases should be exposed to infrared light when receiving sunlight.

For this reason, we should protect ourselves from blue light by wearing red light glasses or living in more natural environments (#456). Numerous studies support the harmfulness of unnatural (outside of appropriate hours) exposure to blue light and LED or artificial light, such as from computers and phones, as they suppress the production of melatonin, which has much more complex functions than simply activating to tell us it is time to sleep.

The goal is to trigger the activity of our mitochondria to generate their own melatonin through red light from the sun, fire or through red light therapy.

Therefore, a valuable recommendation would be:

Change all LED lights in your rooms to red light bulbs to improve sleep quality. Blue light undermines our natural melatonin production and throws off the body's internal biological clock.

Controls daily biological cycles.

This clock is the absolute dictator. The well-known circadian rhythm is governed by our interaction with light.

What happens when your Casio watch fails? Quite simply, you're early or late everywhere. You might show up at work 12 hours late. Or feed your baby after hours. Or try to go to the gym at night when it's already closed.... What I want to point out is that having your biological clock out of sync with the sun also means that you stop functioning.

We are referring to the hormones and neurotransmitters you need to generate or stop generating at the right time, which is as crucial as the food you eat, the air you breathe or the water you drink.

Every time the LED light in your room, the computer screen, cell phone screen or street lamps in the street

•

communicate to your eyes and skin with blue light the current time, your body synchronizes.

The problem lies in the fact that the artificial light tells your body (because of the wavelength of that light) that it is 4 o'clock in the afternoon, but you are actually exposed to it at 8 o'clock in the evening, for example.

Exposing yourself to red light during sunrise hours provides your body with accurate information about the current time. Granted, you can get a little out of sync during the day, but why do everything wrong when we can do some things right? Red light offers benefits beyond what we have explored so far. However, life doesn't give me the time to delve into every one of them.

More and more positive aspects are being revealed:

- Muscular Recovery:
- Decreased pain and inflammation by 70%, according to evidence supported by a meta-analysis, compared to the placebo control group.
- Cognitive improvements observed in all participants.
- Fast and effective recovery from burns.

Is it advisable to purchase a red light luminaire for use in the home?

Is it necessary to purchase a lamp that emits red and infrared light? If you have the time and logistics to greet and bid farewell to the sun, then no, it would not be necessary, although quite beneficial.

Personally, I have acquired two of them, hehe. Although I try to take advantage of the moments of sunrise and sunset depending on the location where I am, it is impossible to ignore the benefits that using the lamps on a daily basis bring me.

Buy **here**

Discount code:

·

D a v i d   B u h n e r

DAVIDBUHNER

Travel and vacation model: Zero by CytoLED .

Giant model for my house: Pentaplex by CytoLED .

I usually take the small device with me when I travel or go on vacation, although it has nothing to do with the sensations and improvements I experience with the large panel I have at home, the sensations are much more intense and after a certain time I start to feel substantially better. If you have a house and you are not a digital nomad or similar I recommend you to buy Pentaplex.

If you live in a big city, it may be a great idea to buy the big lamp. I would recommend you to buy the big lamp if you live in a big city, it can be a great idea to buy the big lamp:

- If you live in a large or small city where buildings block the sun.

- If to see the sunlight you would have to travel far away and travel for 30 minutes, 1 hour, etc.

- Similar situations.

- You live in a place with a climate that is not sunny for all or part of the year, usually in the northern part of the world (most of Europe and the United States, Canada, Russia, large parts of Asia).

- If you live in mountainous areas or in a valley where the light does not reach you well.

- If in your daily life you cannot enjoy the sun due to schedules, working in an office, etc., then you can't enjoy the sun.

After writing this book I have come to the conclusion that most of the benefits of red light are due to the fact that we have a great deficiency of it because of our modern lifestyle.

•

Chapter 2

USES OF A RED LIGHT BULB

Although sunlight is considered the best therapy in many cases, the environment in which we move today does not provide the most conducive logistics to receive its morning benefits and say goodbye to its evening flashes, a practice that would be optimal for our well-being.

Perhaps the view of the sun is obstructed by buildings facing east or west, or perhaps it is necessary to travel long distances to contemplate it, thus sacrificing work time, personal time, etc. In similar situations, I have wondered how to deal with this scenario both in Spain and in other countries around the world.

Currently, there are more than 7,000 scientific studies extolling the benefits of red and infrared light. Despite this, it is undeniable that these research papers leave much to be desired in describing the specific conditions to which the subjects were subjected, conditions that are essential to extrapolate the results to the common user. It would be imperative that they provide detailed details on aspects such as:

- When: Daily frequency, weekly frequency, precise time of day, duration of exposure...
- How: exact configuration of the waves used, recommended protection measures...
- Where: Specific body parts (face, chest, genitals, etc), optimal distance for exposure (1 meter, 5 centimeters, etc).

With the growing impact of the red lamp industry, driven by proven benefits, I am convinced that this boom will not only contribute to price competition, but will also motivate more detailed presentation of scientific evidence. No lies or concealment of data. This, in turn, will allow a more effective extrapolation of the use of these technologies by the user.

When to use a panel and when to use a red light lamp?

•

In anticipation, I have conducted a pragmatic inquiry aimed at those health experts who already own or are contemplating the acquisition of red light bulbs or panels, as I do. The purpose of this inquiry is to clarify any concerns that may arise on this topic.

These are the models I currently use:

https://cytoled.com/products/zero?ref=jzh951y3

- Small model: **CytoLED Zero** .
- Large model that I have in my house: **Pentaplex by CytoLED**.

The large model is much better, although you can't move it from home.

Although it is good to know how these devices work and how to use them, when you receive it at home, do not expect a detailed instruction manual that tells you when and how to use it, since in this field it is often a matter of testing and seeing what works by trial and error.

However, considering the two models I have, the information I have obtained, I have elaborated a small guide that offers guidelines on the appropriate use of these devices, addressing aspects such as temporality, methodology and the ideal place for their application.

How should a red light bulb be used?

I usually use it in bed while waking up or just before going to sleep, also in the bathroom standing up to get the light all over my body.

When during the day can we use the lamps?

In the comprehensive analysis of the extensive evidence from the numerous studies on red light, a notable absence is found in the lack of information regarding the specific time of day when the infrared light therapies were performed, which is truly surprising.

Although we can infer that, given the common pattern in many studies where subjects attend clinics Monday through Friday, until approximately 6 p.m., this allows us to speculate that it is likely that we can employ our lamp at any time of the day to obtain the benefits mentioned in these studies.

•

Importantly, some studies highlight the importance of marking the time of day when therapies were performed, incorporating control and placebo groups. One example is a study with athletes who had red light applied to half of their body during the night, with a duration of 30 minutes.

However, it is crucial to be aware of different practices, as some people, instead of directing light to lower parts of the body, apply it to the face during the night. This, paradoxically, can result in overstimulation, as even red light, if its brightness and intensity are too high, can inhibit melatonin production, making it difficult to fall asleep.

I personally use red light therapy in the morning after waking up or before going to bed in order to simulate a sunrise and sunset in my body.

How many minutes are adequate?

In most red light fixtures, the right thing to do would be to use it for about 5-20 minutes, with a distance of about 50-60 cm. However, in the smaller device I own, this range extends to 10-40 minutes, as it has a lower wattage. In contrast, with the large panel, I usually run sessions of about 15 minutes, typically.

How many sessions per week are appropriate?

It is completely feasible to use it once a day to maintain overall good health. Personally I usually do a session when I wake up and at bedtime, which adds up to a total of 2 a day, although sometimes I do up to 3 or even 4.

It is important to note that it is necessary to allow at least one hour between each session.

Where to use a red and infrared light bulb

Adequate distance

According to studies, the ideal point to use the lamp is at a distance of 40, 50 or 60 centimeters, which is the ideal point for the red and infrared NIR rays to be dispersed evenly throughout the body. However, I have to admit that I simply stick the lamp to my body, obtaining good results.

In case you are at a greater distance, it would be necessary to extend the time of the session to be really effective. In the case of my larger panel, for example, even if I were 2 meters away, I would have to multiply the duration of my session by about 4 to

•

maintain the desired effectiveness.

On the other hand, using my smaller lamp, I could stay up to 1 meter away for effective results. However, it would be necessary to increase the duration of my session 2.5 times to achieve the desired effectiveness.

That is, with the smaller lamp I would stand at a distance of 50 centimeters, which would be about the length of my arm.

What part of you needs to be exposed to light therapy?

It is more beneficial to apply the light to large areas of the body. With the large panel, it practically covers me completely, while with the smaller lamp, when I take it on a trip, I concentrate on my stomach, chest or even my back. If I do the session in the morning, I also make sure it reaches the face and scalp.

Should I point the red, infrared light at my testicles - is it good or bad?

Many male readers may be wondering if they can expose their testicles to light. Yes, there are studies that suggest an increase in testosterone levels and libido after red light therapy.

However, it is important and necessary to exercise caution, as I have found studies indicating possible damage to the testes of rats due to inordinate overexposure to red light.

It should be noted that these studies do not provide adequate information on the dose used or the parameters established. In other words, we cannot determine whether very high doses were used, excessive doses were used, or whether the rat testes were overheated in a manner similar to the way they would be heated if you put them in a frying pan.

In my perspective, although I have observed numerous positive anecdotes related to increased testosterone and libido through this therapy, the paucity of solid evidence urges us to be cautious and avoid excessive exposure in that area.

I want to clarify that I am not issuing recommendations. Each individual is responsible for his or her decisions. I personally limit the exposure of my testicles to red and infrared light.

•

David Buhner

Proper way to use the red light bulb

1. **Timer panel:** will give you important data about the timer configuration, such as what type of timer configuration have you chosen? How many minutes and seconds are left? The first two digits indicate the minutes, while the other two show the seconds, easy and obvious. It is relevant to note that when you turn on the panel, it will automatically show the timer activated (set by default to 10 minutes) at least that's how this model works. If the display shows "FF:FF", it means that the timer is deactivated and the lamp will remain on indefinitely, at least until you turn it off or activate the timer.

2. **Infrared light on the display:** signals that the 850nm illumination is operating at maximum.

3. **Red light:** when you see the light indicator at 660nm, you know it's doing its job.

4. **Time control:** this little button is the key to manage the timer. Press it to turn it on and off according to your needs. The trick is that you can set it up to 30 minutes. And you know, if it's not running, the display will show "FF:FF".

5. **Light wave type selector:** with this small button, you have

control over what type of light you want the panel to emit. You can choose between red light, infrared light, or even both at the same time. If you haven't pressed the little button, it is factory set to illuminate with both. If you touch it once = you turn off both. Another tap = NIR (850nm) infrared light only. Another tap and only the red light (660nm) will turn on. Tap it one more time and you are back to the combination of both wavelengths. My recommendation is to keep all types of lights active each time you use it, so you can get the maximum benefits.

6. **Time Adder (Timer):** With this button we can extend the timer time by 1 minute for each "click". If the time remaining on the timer is not an exact minute, the panel will adjust the minutes to the value closest to the current time. Instead of pressing the button repeatedly, you can press and hold the button if you prefer. If you hit the button when the time has reached zero, it will reset the timer to 10 minutes, which is the default value.

7. **Time subtractor (Timer):** By pressing the "Minus" button, you will decrease the timer time (if it is running) by 1 minute for each time you press it. Its operation is similar to the "Plus" button (6), but here, if you press it when there is only 1 minute left, instead of going to zero, it will take you directly to 30 minutes on the timer.

•

Excessive exposure

Maintaining a balance with red light is key, not too little and not too much. From the info I have reviewed, saturating yourself with red light (in amounts greater than recommended) does not appear to be harmful to the body, just less effective.

It is crucial to consider that our different tissues are at different depths in the body. So, to get the optimal dose of red and infrared light in one tissue, it may be necessary for another tissue to receive a little more. In that sense, it makes sense that problems can arise.

Although when it comes to the body as a whole rather than specific tissues, there is less information on how it actually responds to certain doses. It is a less explored terrain.

Should I protect myself with glasses?

What happens if I put the red or infrared light in my eyes? With the lamp you will receive the lamp with goggles included as part of the package. Normally light is not a problem, but if the light in your eyes has too much intensity, or if the light is in your eyes for too long, this could lead to a thermal effect. And that will make our eyes more sensitive, it's as simple as that. It's like if you stand in front of a 'lit' fireplace, this will not have in principle any negative effect on your eyes, but if you stand one centimeter away from the fire for 1 hour you will obviously have problems, it's just common sense.

When you close your eyes, much of the light bounces off your skin. This phenomenon can be quite significant, providing protection against excessive levels and effectively scattering light. This is recommended, and your skin's natural detectors in your eyelids will let you know when it's time to stop.

Of course, it all depends on who you are and what you look like - not all bodies and eyes are the same. If you are prone to experiencing eye discomfort very easily, whether due to photosensitivity, migraines or other visual complications, it makes sense to consider wearing glasses or some kind of protection to ensure greater comfort - it's just common sense.

Some may have read somewhere that red light can trigger cataracts, but if you do a little research you will realize that these are just unfounded rumors. They have even mentioned something about the need for sunscreen during red light sessions, which is totally absurd. These are totally false stories.

•

At the opposite end of these stories is some research that points to visual improvements in those who have been exposed to the lower levels of infrared light emitted by such lamps. Younger individuals barely noticed significant changes, while those with more experience experienced a 20% increase in color perception and an improvement in the sensitivity of the rods, which are photoreceptors in the retina.

There are guidelines, such as those established by the International Electrotechnical Commission, which indicate that, in order to safeguard the health of our eyes, the recommended limit would be 57 milliwatts per square centimeter for less than 100 seconds. It is important to take into consideration that these guidelines refer to directly observing that light source during the aforementioned period and not when looking at it indirectly.

When we uncovered the chicanery of some manufacturers of red and infrared light lamps. It is seen in analysis that the eye can tolerate up to 80 mW/cm2 for less than 30 seconds before thermal damage begins to manifest itself. And what is the connection to the manufacturers? Well, it turns out to be crucial in every respect. Otherwise, we would all end up visually exhausted after a red light session, or worse with eye damage.

Companies claiming that the radiation from their models exceeds 100 mW/cm2 should be transparent and provide an explanation of how they are misleading us:

- Do you sell lights that are harmful to the human eye?
- Or are they lying about their products?

There are no other options.

Most likely the second possibility is the correct one and we are being deceived by these companies. That is why in my list of the leading brands of red light bulbs, I have not suggested any of those that seem to tell lies. If we realize that we are being fooled on one thing, it would not be surprising if we are being fooled on other things as well.

It is paradoxical that protective goggles are provided with the lamp. Also, many times if you test them with a meter, those goggles do not offer any kind of protection against infrared light. So why do they include them, what is going on, is it safe or not, it is obviously better not to even use the brands that have this kind of strategy. I repeat do not use under any context any product or service of this type of companies or brands.

At the conclusion of the day, all the lamp brands end up providing you with a pair of those effect glasses so you have your placebo effect, simply because it's common practice, and none of them want to be the brand that gets left out of the trend. It's a matter of marketing.

In short, I:

- I never or almost never wear glasses.
- Or I simply close my eyelids so that the heat or thermal effect does not affect my eyes.
- Or I look around without looking directly into the lamps.

I also often do a combination of several strategies.

C H A P T E R 3

Which red light bulb to purchase?

Most brands lie to you by 90%. The red and infrared light lamp is nothing more than the modern substitute for the infrared and red waves emitted by the sun, especially during sunrise and sunset.

Is it essential for staying healthy? While sun exposure is, owning such a lamp is questionable.

David Buhner

I have 2 lamps, but I would only recommend them only to those people who cannot make the effort or lack the logistics necessary to contemplate the sun during sunrise and sunset.

Many people are surprised that the sun is not only beneficial for vitamin D absorption.

There are many studies online about red or infrared light, but it is really difficult to know which is the best red light on the market.

I currently have 2 lamp models, the reason I purchased 2 and not 1 or 3 was because I contacted all the companies that market red and infrared light panels, asking some specific questions about the lamps, after doing this I got a list of 3 brands that did not lie to me or misrepresent their answers, evidencing their commitment to scientific and commercial integrity rather than trying to sell you something using unlawful or immoral methods.

David Buhner

What is a red light bulb and what is its function?

The red and infrared light lamp (or panel) is an electronic device that replaces sunlight. We use the term "lamp" to refer to smaller models and red light "panel" when referring to a larger and heavier design (one meter or even more), which when turned on covers most of the surface of the body.

Just as when we mention "red light" we refer to both red and infrared light, when we say "lamp" today I refer to both the "panel" and the red light lamp. These are technological devices that emit wavelengths between 660 and 850 nanometers, a range where light has been found to provide therapeutic benefits.

It is essential to clarify that simply changing the color of the light bulbs in your home to red is not enough. Red light offers clear and recognized benefits for sleep and other aspects that we will discuss later, but right now we are talking about devices technologically designed to emit infrared radiation (which is radiation not visible to the human eye), mimicking that provided by the sun. These radiations many of us overlook due to our routines during dawn and dusk (times when they are more abundant).

In recent months, I have dedicated myself to exposing my body, especially my chest and abs, not only during peak UVB hours to get vitamin D from the sun, but also during sunrises to absorb more infrared light, and I have also exposed myself as much as possible to the evening light, although it has not been easy.

Which lamp should you buy?

What did I consider before selecting a red light and infrared lamp model?

1. Radiation (a point where most manufacturers are not honest or at least not very transparent): Electromagnetic radiation emissions, their health implications, etc.

2. The possibility of choosing the light frequencies in a specific way.

3. The presence of flicker.

4. The angle of the red and infrared lights.

5. Other additional factors.

With an irradiation of less than 100 mW/cm2.

The first aspect to consider is irradiation, as this is where 90% of manufacturers deceive us, something immoral, illegal, etc. that should always make us discard the brand. If they deceive us in this aspect, we could be acquiring a device that emits red light but without any therapeutic benefits. They would be giving us something different from what we are looking for.

To better understand irradiance and what values to look for, we can narrow down our list to just a few trusted brands.

In more technical language, "irradiance" or "power density" is the light energy on a surface, i.e. the power reaching our skin, measured in milliwatts per square centimeter (mW/cm2). This irradiance determines whether the light from the lamp can penetrate deep enough to stimulate our cells.

It is crucial to keep in mind that, while it is true that without sufficient irradiance we do not get adequate benefits, manufacturers and companies selling these lamps sometimes manipulate the intensity numbers to create the illusion of guaranteed benefits. However, in the case of red light, there is a sweet spot, because dosage is the key. Not too much and not too little.

It is true that if you purchase such a lamp and it is not bright enough, you will need to expose yourself longer. However, the opposite is also true. If it is too powerful, it could heat up your body cells too much.

Many will be wondering why the model I have chosen has less power than other lamps of the same size on the market. It's not that it's less powerful, it's that it's as powerful as it should be, and the other brands are lying.

You will find models with more than 100 mW/cm2, more than 200 mW/cm2, etc, why buy a 60 mW/cm2, because it is simple, many studies show that a lamp of more than 100 mW/cm2 used on your skin does not really have many benefits compared to one of 60 mW/cm2, moreover a device of more than 100 mW/cm2 can be dangerous.

These brands have evaluated their lamps and panels using solar energy meters, devices to measure the spectrum of sunlight. These devices as they are designed provide false values, up to 4 times higher. Theoretically they are not lying, but they are deceiving us.

Brands and companies that claim on their websites and social networks that their lamps radiate +100mW/cm2 are not only questionable, but also not recommended at all. Not only because they deceive us (and who knows what else they lie about), but because it is crucial to plot irradiance over a wide range of distances instead of providing a single measurement. In this way, we can know precisely how much light energy we receive.

When you are shopping for an infrared and red light lamp or panel, you will notice that there are larger models and smaller models. That is, the larger models are much more productive. For this reason, I have a small one for traveling and a larger five-foot panel in my house.

But maybe you want to buy a lamp or panel not for general benefits as I did, but to perform infrared therapy on specific parts of the skin, bones, muscles, etc. In this case, it is logically more than enough to choose the smallest model you can afford and that is of good quality to direct all the light to that part instead of focusing on the irradiation.

Particular light frequencies

In relation to this aspect, the second criterion for selecting our lamp is to consider not only the light frequencies to which we expose ourselves, but also the ability to choose specifically between them according to our specific daily objectives. The benefits of red light lie in the range between 660 and 850 nanometers, and these lamps and panels have been designed precisely to cover this particular spectrum.

Visible red light of 660 nanometers is much more suitable for the treatment of superficial tissues, such as the skin, as it penetrates much less deeply. On the other hand, non-visible infrared light of 850 nanometers is more suitable for the treatment of somewhat deeper tissues, such as muscles, cells and various functions, as it penetrates more deeply. While the red light that is visible to the human eye is absorbed by the first layers of the skin, generating cellular responses, infrared light reaches even further, penetrating through all layers of the skin to the muscles, bones and of course the external organs.

In most red light lamps and panels, such as the ones I own, 660 nm and 850 nm wavelengths are emitted in a balanced manner. The former is visible to the human eye, while the latter, although not visible, penetrates much deeper. However, the ratio is not 50/50; when choosing a red light lamp, it is critical to ensure that for every 850 nm emission, 1.3 times as many wavelengths are emitted at 660 nm.

It may be beneficial to select a model that allows you to choose each range independently. For example, you can opt for infrared light only and not red in certain situations, it all depends on what you want the light for whether to repair tissue, improve cognition, reduce wrinkles, lose subcutaneous fat, stimulate collagen, prevent sunburn, increase melatonin and improve sleep, as well as for muscle recovery.

As I usually seek to improve my overall health, I tend to use all the wavelengths available to me. Among the lamps I have, the small one I take on a trip does not allow me to customize the types of light, but the larger panel I have at home, with a length of 1.5 meters, does give me the possibility to independently select each type of light, focusing on specific benefits according to what I am interested in at that specific moment.

It should have a density of about 60 J/cm2.

Another aspect to take into account is the density of the light that these lamps emit, what is light density, it would be the amount of light energy that the cells receive. In other words, how many cells are you affecting and to what extent. If previously we examined the intensity with which you are impacting them, now we focus on how many cells you are affecting, that is, the number of cells.

This density is measured in Joules per square centimeter (J/cm2), not in calories, not in photons or in mW/cm2, how many Joules should the perfect lamp have for home infrared therapy to work well? According to studies, around 4-5 J/cm2 per session offers the best benefits.

The number of Joules that provide no improvement is above 50 in some studies. This, in biology, is known as hormesis, where a mild exposure to a stressor greatly strengthens the body's defenses against much stronger stressors.

And where can we look at these Joules? The manufacturers usually do not provide this information and it is not visible anywhere on the device or in the instructions. Obtaining Joules is based on the duration of the treatment, there is a formula that we could use to make the calculation, but it is not necessary to use it, nor to know it, just follow more or less the table below:

	Infrared light	Red light
Distance: 10cm Duration: 10m	33 J/cm2	24 J/cm2
Distance: 20cm Duration: 20m	24 J/cm2	16.8 J/cm2
Distance: 30cm Duration: 30m	16.2 J/cm2	10.2 J/cm2

I put this table here so that you know what you are really buying, but it is not particularly important.

The orientation of the red and infrared light beam.

Some manufacturers often indicate that the angle of the light can be quite an important factor if you want to get the maximum benefit from the lamp, red and infrared and this is something to keep in mind that we should not overlook. For example, when mentioning a LED beam with a large angle which are those light bulbs that claim to have a significant angle, such as 60° or more), this implies that the light will scatter very quickly, too quickly and will cover a larger area on the body, but at the same time it will lose intensity as it moves away, reducing its health effects.

At the other end of the scale, a somewhat narrower angle means less coverage (less body part), but the intensity would be much more concentrated even at considerably greater distances. The natural angle of most LEDs is around 120 degrees, although using reflectors and lenses, we can adjust it to our liking with more conventional angles such as: 90°, 60°, 30°, and even 10°.

It is important to note that, while this factor has its relevance, beam angle is not the most crucial metric nor the first one you would consider when looking for an effective light bulb for red light and infrared light therapy, but this is something you can use as an indicator of the quality of the product you are buying, as 90% of manufacturers do not include this information in the specifications.

When you review the descriptions of many of the models of red and infrared light therapy lamps, you will see that they often state that it is mandatory to be close or very close to the LED to get the best or at least effective results. In essence, they are making a generalization based on the fact that most LED lights have a wide angle, although there are now many models that concentrate the beam at much narrower angles.

The most optimal option is when the lamp has a wide or high beam angle, which implies that we must be close to obtain benefits. On the other hand, if the light beam is concentrated at a reduced angle, it is advisable to maintain a certain distance.

The lamp and panel I own both have 60° angles, so I tend to use them close together, which is quite comforting and comfortable. A fundamental aspect for any brand or model would be to share a chart with the intensity at the recommended distance. This allows us to clearly and optimally determine from what distance to perform red and infrared light therapy, considering intensity, coverage and of course comfort.

Despite reviewing all the available evidence, I have not found any specific studies on beam angles in red light therapy. However, I do not rule out that they will start to emerge soon, and to that it is more than clear that the overall benefits are clearly real and we can now delve much deeper into the details.

If we apply the logic regarding intensity, coverage and irradiance, the beam angle would be a very relevant component only if you want to treat a specific tissue or perform therapy on a specific part of the body. But for now, we are looking for devices that report the effective intensity at various distances from the device. This saves us from having to perform complex calculations to determine angles and distances.

When selecting one of these devices, I usually pay attention mainly to the minimum distance recommended for use by the manufacturer. The closer we are during therapy, the less relevant the angle will be, but it is important to be careful not to be "too close".

Machines must not pulsing

You may find models that offer the option of pulsing. This feature involves very fast switching on and off of the lamps, measured in Hz(Hertz). In other words, if we say 10 Hz, the light turns on and off 10 times per second on average.

However, we must be extremely clear that this function is rather pseudoscience, i.e. "science" without scientific evidence. The evidence so far does not support this feature. I quote: "it was impossible to establish a significant correlation between pulse rate and pathological condition, due to the great variety and disparity of data. As for other pulse parameters, they were deficient or inconclusive".

Therefore, if we come across a brand that includes this function, we should be quite skeptical, as it lacks scientific backing. It is likely that they are incorporating it just to differentiate themselves in the market and to have a good marketing, nothing more. This should make us doubt the brand and the model. We must also be aware that this will also mean a higher price than the competition that does not have the pulsing function.

This type of rather dishonest practices can also be observed in the information on the emitted irradiation or in the inclusion of "protective" glasses, aspects that I will refute later on, since they do not fulfill any useful function despite the fact that all brands include them.

No flicker free effect

An important consideration when choosing a lamp is to check if the brand name mentions that the model is "flicker free". Flicker refers to the on and off of the LED light in these lamps or panels. Imagine a party with lights constantly flickering on and off.

Although flickering occurs so fast that the average human eye does NOT perceive it consciously, it can affect us on a subconscious level, which is certainly the major difference with the pulsing effect. Since the popularization of LED light, many technologies related to this light source show this characteristic phenomenon. Sensitive people may experience some health problems, from migraines to panic attacks, dizziness, nausea and other symptoms, although extreme situations are rare.

Flicker is not unimportant, as it can cause significant long-term effects such as photosensitivity, chronic migraines, chronic fatigue, anxiety and depression. Although there is little specific information on the flicker effect in red light and infrared therapies, it is essential to look for lamps that are flicker-free. If you really want to do a lot of research and make sure that the lamp is flicker-free, there are devices called spectrometers that can measure the flickering of a red and infrared light lamp.

These spectrometers usually provide quite detailed data, such as the flicker hertz (the frequency with which the light changes) and the exact flicker percentage (the variation in brightness). For example, 2 lamps with 100

Hertz may have different flicker percentages, with the one with the higher percentage being more problematic.

If you have already purchased a panel and are not experiencing significant discomfort, it may not be necessary to return it, considering the cost of these devices. It is important to keep in mind that most flicker-related problems are chronic and result from constant exposure, as in the case of office workers who have been under fluorescent lights for years.

In addition, during lamp exposure, we generally do not perform cognitively demanding tasks. It is essential to distinguish between flicker and light pulse, where the latter is simply a controlled flicker of light, pulsing at a certain frequency.

Reduced levels of electromagnetic radiation

Finally, after having taken into account all of the above, something that I consider of utmost importance and is one of the first things I check is... that the device has a low electromagnetic radiation emission.

If the brand is a manufacturer committed to science and not pseudoscience, marketing or money, it will have designed the lamp so that it can be used in hospital and clinical environments, where electromagnetic radiation levels must be kept strictly low to avoid interference with other wave-sensitive equipment.

Personally, I would find it counterintuitive and even an absolute contradiction to purchase an additional electronic device that promised numerous benefits, but at the same time was exposing me to radiation, being aware of the effects that electromagnetic waves can have on health.

But... What is the best red light bulb?

Considering all of the above, I present to you the type of red light lamp I finally decided to purchase, as well as the full body panel.

- Discount code: PON DISCOUNT CODE

- Travel lamp: Zero by CytoLED (highly recommended, don't forget to use the discount code).
- Large lamp that I use at home: Pentaplex from CytoLED (approximately 1,700 € without taking into account the coupon).
- Remark: Although I take the smaller size Zero lamp with me everywhere I go, I miss the sensations that the giant panel provides at each session due to its higher intensity level. If you own a house or do not move often you should buy it, I recommend without hesitation the Pentaplex model.

Why did I choose this brand for both the lamp and the panel?

Well, it happens to be one of only three brands (and the only one in Europe) that offers all of the features detailed above:

- With scientific integrity (no deception in irradiation).
- The light intensity (irradiance) is powerful enough to provide us with 17 to 73 mv/cm2 (milliwatts per square centimeter) at most.
- The light frequency ranges from 660 to 850 nanometers (red light).
- Low electromagnetic radiation and no flicker.

Note on affiliation: All red light and infrared companies have affiliate and referral programs (they create coupons so that if you refer someone, they pay you a commission). Some offer sky-high commissions, but that doesn't mean their products are the best (the end customer ends up paying the price). That's why the lamp models I have selected have been chosen based on the model and brand, not on their affiliate program.

Prices start in the low hundreds and the best red light lamp models are found in Europe, USA and Australia. I do not recommend Aliexpress because, in testing them with specific questions, I found that some sellers lie in their specifications and answers to sell the product at all costs.

The first one I bought was from the United States, but customs wanted me to pay 450€, so I decided not to pay them and return the product.

Brands shipping from Europe

- **Differentiated shipping and invoicing:** If you want to save money as a company or freelancer, some suppliers issue invoices with a different address or country than the actual location where the product is received. While others require that both the billing and shipping addresses match.

- **Flicker:** There is no invisible flicker to the human eye.

- **Electromagnetic radiation:** Lamps and panels have been designed considering electromagnetic waves for health.

.

CytoLED

- Origin: The Netherlands
- Deception in irradiation: No
- Flicker: No
- Electromagnetic radiation: No
- Shipping and invoicing in different countries: Yes

NanoROTLicht

- Origin: Germany
- Deception in irradiation: Yes
- Shipping and invoicing in different countries: Yes

LumiRed

- Origin: Ireland
- Deception in irradiation: Yes
- Shipping and invoicing in different countries: Yes

MitoLight

- Origin: Czech Republic

	• Deception in irradiation: no
	• Shipping and invoicing in different countries: Yes
	• Origin: Germany
Aurora Red Light	• Deception in irradiation: Yes
	• Shipping and invoicing in different countries: Yes
	• Origin: Finland
Innolux	• Deception in irradiation: Yes
	• Shipping and invoicing in different countries: Yes
	• Origin: Finland
CuRed	• Deception in irradiation: Yes
	• Shipping and invoicing in different countries: Yes

Brands that ship internationally

- **Customs:** All these companies are subject to customs duties and taxes upon receipt of the lamp.

- **Customized" invoice**: A few companies agree to generate a "customized invoice", indicating that the value of the device is less than the actual amount you have paid. For example, if you've paid €1,000, the enclosed invoice may specify a value of €200, for the purpose of reducing customs costs. It is not legal and I do not recommend it obviously, but many people pay attention to this, obviously if your order is lost by accident or not the compensation will be much less, this is very unlikely but it can happen.

GembaRed
- Origin: United States
- Deception on irradiation: No
- Shipping and invoicing in different countries: Yes
- Personalized invoice:No

EMR-TEK
- Origin: Canada
- Deception in irradiation: Yes
- Shipping and invoicing in different countries: Yes
- Customized invoice: No

MitoGen
- Origin: Australia
- Deception on irradiation: No
- Shipping and invoicing in different countries: Yes
- Customized invoice: No

Infraredi
- Origin: Australia

- Deception in irradiation: Yes

- Shipping and invoicing in different countries: Yes

- Customized invoice: Yes
- Origin: United States

Joovv

- Shipping and invoicing in different countries: Yes

- Customized invoice: No
- Origin: United States

MitoRedLight

- Shipping and invoicing in different countries: Yes

- Customized invoice: No
- Origin: Australia

Bon Charge

- Shipping and invoicing in different countries: Yes

- Customized invoice: No
- Origin: United States

Platinum Therapy Lights

- Shipping and invoicing in different countries: Yes

- Customized invoice: No
- Origin: United Kingdom

Red Light Rising

- Shipping and invoicing in different countries: Yes

- Customized invoice: No

David Buhner

Sources, references and notes

- 1

Gavish L, Houreld NN. Therapeutic Efficacy of Home-Use Photobiomodulation Devices: A Systematic Literature Review. Photobiomodul Photomed Laser Surg. 2019 Jan;37(1):4-16. doi: 10.1089/photob.2018.4512. PMID: 31050938.

- 2

Barolet D. Light-emitting diodes (LEDs) in dermatology. Semin Cutan Med Surg. 2008 Dec;27(4):227-238.

- 3

Huang YY, Chen AC, Carroll JD, Hamblin MR. Biphasic dose response in low level light therapy. Dose Response. 2009 Sep 1;7(4):358-83. doi: 10.2203/dose-response.09-027.Hamblin. PMID: 20011653; PMCID: PMC2790317.

- 4

Lee SY, Park KH, Choi JW, Kwon JK, Lee DR, Shin MS, Lee JS, You CE, Park MY. A prospective, randomized, placebo-controlled, double-blinded, and split-face clinical study on LED phototherapy for skin rejuvenation: clinical, profilometric, histologic, ultrastructural, and biochemical evaluations and comparison of three different treatment settings. J Photochem Photobiol B. 2007 Jul 27;88(1):51-67. doi: 10.1016/j.jphotobiol.2007.04.008. Epub 2007 May 1. PMID: 17566756.

- 5

Gavish L, Houreld NN. Therapeutic Efficacy of Home-Use Photobiomodulation Devices: A Systematic Literature Review. Photobiomodul Photomed Laser Surg. 2019 Jan;37(1):4-16. doi: 10.1089/photob.2018.4512. PMID: 31050938.

- 6

Avci P, Gupta A, Sadasivam M, Vecchio D, Pam Z, Pam N, Hamblin MR. Low-level laser (light) therapy (LLLT) in skin: stimulating, healing, restoring. Semin Cutan Med Surg. 2013 Mar;32(1):41-52. PMID: 24049929; PMCID: PMC4126803.

- 7

Hashmi JT, Huang YY, Sharma SK, Kurup DB, De Taboada L, Carroll JD, Hamblin MR. Effect of pulsing in low-level light therapy. Lasers Surg Med. 2010 Aug;42(6):450-66. doi: 10.1002/lsm.20950. PMID: 20662021; PMCID: PMC2933784.

- 8

Karanovic O, Thabet M, Wilson HR, Wilkinson F. Detection and discrimination of flicker contrast in migraine. Cephalalgia. 2011 Apr;31(6):723-36. doi: 10.1177/0333102411398401. PMID: 21493642; PMCID: PMC3571449.

- 9

IEEE Recommended Practices for Modulating Current in High-Brightness LEDs for Mitigating Health Risks to Viewers

- 10

Fisher RS, Acharya JN, Baumer FM, French JA, Parisi P, Solodar JH, Szaflarski JP, Thio LL, Tolchin B, Wilkins AJ, Kasteleijn-Nolst Trenité D. Visually sensitive seizures: An updated review by the Epilepsy Foundation. Epilepsia. 2022 Apr;63(4):739-768. doi: 10.1111/epi.17175. epub 2022 Feb 7. PMID: 35132632.

- 11

Radford B, Bartholomew R. Pokémon contagion: photosensitive epilepsy or mass psychogenic illness? South Med J. 2001 Feb;94(2):197-204. PMID: 11235034.

- 12

Salet N, Visser M, Stam C, Smulders YM. Stroboscopic light effects during electronic dance music festivals and photosensitive epilepsy: a cohort study and case report. BMJ Open. 2019 Jun 11;9(6):e023442. doi: 10.1136/bmjopen-2018-023442. PMID: 31186244; PMCID: PMC6585837.

- 13

Kennedy A, Murray WS. The effects of flicker on eye movement control. Q J Exp Psychol A. 1991 Feb;43(1):79-99. doi: 10.1080/14640749108401000. PMID: 2017572.

- 14

Kennedy A, Murray WS. The effects of flicker on eye movement control. Q J Exp Psychol A. 1991 Feb;43(1):79-99. doi: 10.1080/14640749108401000. PMID: 2017572.

- 15

"IEEE Recommended Practices for Modulating Current in High-Brightness LEDs for Mitigating Health Risks to Viewers," in IEEE Std 1789-2015 , vol., no., pp.1-80, 5 June 2015.

- 16

IEEE Recommended Practices for Modulating Current in High-Brightness LEDs for Mitigating Health Risks to Viewers .

ABOUT THE AUTHOR

David buhner is one of the most prolific authors in existence today, he has written several books on health, many of his works have been translated into several languages: English, French, German, Japanese, Portuguese, Dutch, etc.

FINAL WORDS

Thank you for reading and trusting me as an author, this book has cost a lot to make, if you liked the book please support me with a positive opinion where you bought the book: amazon, etc, if you have obtained this book by non-legal means, I hold absolutely no grudge and I hope you know how to take advantage of the knowledge that I exposed here. Consider buying the book in paper, as well as posting a positive review if you consider it.